**Fadama CONDE**

**Experience of the urology department of HMIMV Rabat:**

*ABBREVIATIONS*

*AA: arteries*

*AFU :*  *Association* française d'urologie *IR* : Index of vascular resistance

IS : Arterial insufficiency

*MRI: magnetic resonance imaging FCC: fracture of the corpus cavernosum*

*PGE1: Prostaglandin E1*

*PSV: peak systolic arterial velocity EDV: end-diastolic arterial velocity SS:*

*sympathetic system*

*SPS: parasympathetic system*

*UCRM: urinary retrograde urethrocystography Vv: veins*

# CONTENTS

# *INTRODUCTION*

## *General*

Fracture of the penis is a uro-andrological emergency that occurs in the majority of cases on an erect penis (*thickness of the albuginea at rest= 3mm, during erection the thickness decreases to 0.25 -0.50mm)*; this variation leads to a drop in resistance within the albuginea to sudden overpressure events, causing it to rupture.

The most frequently reported etiology is the coite faux pas, among many others.

Diagnosis is clinical, and relies on a range of arguments gathered through careful questioning and physical examination (cracking, detumescence, hematoma, pain at the end, producing an aubergine-like appearance). The occurrence of hematuria requires a search for urethral involvement.

Secondarily complemented by ultrasound in the first instance, given availability in the emergency department, followed by MRI and cavernography, depending on the authors.

Management should be carried out as early as possible to avoid post-operative complications.

It relies on surgery, with either a coronal incision that risks skin necrosis, or an elective incision that risks missing certain lesions.

*In the light of the data collected in the literature, our series analyzes the epidemiological, diagnostic, therapeutic, evolutionary and postoperative follow-up aspects of a retrospective study of six (06) cases at HMIMV Rabat over a period of three years.*

## *A- History*

The notion of fractured corpora cavernosa dates back 1,000 years, when Abul Kacem wrote of a fracture of the penis due to damage to the corpora cavernosa (1,2).

The first observation was made in 1787 by Trye (3). Other publications include :

- JP Franck in 1808 (4)
- V. Mott in 1847(5)


Rupture of the corpus cavernosum was first described in 1925(7), followed by REDIRE in 1926 and Puigvert and Macias 1946(8).
- Thompson in 1954 (9) published new observations a n d  agreed that the lesion mainly concerned the corpora cavernosa.
- In 1957, Fenestron (10) published 18 cases and noted that

The risk of urethral damage is very high when flexion occurs at the penoscrotal angle, and very low when it occurs distally;

The direction of torsion determines the location of the lesion.

As far as treatment is concerned, this condition has undergone considerable change over the years.

The first case of surgical treatment was reported by Fetter in 1936.

In 1957, Fenestron (10) surgically repaired an old sequela, ushering in a new era in this field.

Nowadays, most authors agree that surgery is the only way to avoid complications compared to medical treatments.


## *B- ANATOMICAL REMINDER*

The penis is the male organ of copulation, but also the terminal organ of micturition. Located in front of the pubic symphysis. It is crossed by the urethra, which opens at its distal end via the urethral meatus.

We distinguish :

## *B-a  ENVELOPES*

1- A thick albuginea surrounds each erectile body.

2- The deep fascia of the penis, which surrounds a large cellular space that explains the possibility of the sheath "sliding" over the erectile formations.

3- The dartos (superficial fascia of the penis). 3- The skin or sheath of the penis

### B-b : Means of fixation of the penis :

The body is held in place by its continuity with the root and by the suspensory and funsiform ligaments, which comprise. :

*1. The suspensory ligament of the penis*: Triangular. It arises in front of the pubic symphysis, spreading out and dividing into two blades that attach on either side of the corpus cavernosum, on the deep fascia of the penis.

*2. The fundiform ligament of the penis:* arises from the lower part of the linea alba, then crosses the mound of the pubis. It divides into two blades that pass on either side of the suspensory ligament of the penis.

*Configuration :*

The penis consists of two topographically and functionally distinct parts:

- A)The root, hidden in the perineum and fixed ;
- B )The body, visible and mobile.

*A. The root of the penis*: Located in the superficial space of the perineum, above the scrotum. It comprises the two pillars and the bulb of the penis.

1. Pillars of the penis: These represent the posterior parts of the corpora cavernosa. Each pillar attaches to an ischiopubic branch in front of the ischial tuberosity, and to the lower fascia of the urogenital diaphragm. Surrounded by the ischiocavernosus muscle.

2. 2. The bulb of the penis: Represents the posterior part of the spongy body. Attaches to the underside of the perineal membrane. It is covered by the bulbo spongiosus muscle.

It is pyriform and median. The urethra passes through its deep surface, 1 or 2 cm from its posterior end, and more laterally, the ducts of the bulbo urethral glands.

*B.*    *The body of the penis:* when flaccid, it lies under the pubic symphysis in front of the scrotum, and when erect, in front of the pubic symphysis:

-    Its shape is cylindrical, more or less flattened sagittally, with an anterior face or dorsum of the penis, a posterior face or urethral face, and a swollen free end, the glans.

-    Dimensions Highly variable in adults, the body measures :

➢    In its flaccid state, it measures 10 to 12 cm in length and 8 to 9 cm in circumference.

➢    When erect: 16 to 18 cm long, 11 to 12 cm in circumference (3 to 4 cm in diameter). Anatomy of the male genitalia: The Verge


## C.    Structure of the penis:

The penis is made up o f three cylinders of erectile tissue: 1- the two corpora cavernosa; 2- the corpus spongiosum and 3- the glans.

These erectile bodies, isolated in the root, gather under the pubis to help form the body of the penis.

### 1.    *Corpus cavernosum:*
-    ***Histologically,*** *the corpora cavernosa are made up of connective tissue, numerous elastic fibers and smooth muscle bundles that form the sinusoidal or blood spaces: virtual spaces filled by helical arteries and evacuated by emissary veins.*

-    ***Anatomically speaking,*** the corpora cavernosa are narrowed and conical at the ends, and lean medially against the body. They are separated by the septum of the penis.  They delimit two longitudinal grooves:
One, upper, for the deep dorsal vein of the penis, on the back of the penis. The lower one for the spongy body, on the urethral surface.


### 2.    *The spongy body:*
-    ***Histologically,*** *the spongy tissue is made up of cavernous-type tissue, but is less developed than that of the corpus cavernosum proper. Its albuginea is also thinner, with less abundant elastic and muscular fibers.*
-    ***Anatomically speaking,*** the corpus spongiosum originates behind the bulb.

It continues forward through the glans. It surrounds the spongy urethra and runs in the lower longitudinal groove of the corpora cavernosa. The urethra penetrates the corpus spongiosum at the level of the upper surface of the bulb.


3.    *Acorn*:
•      The free end of the penis is covered by the foreskin. It is conical, smooth and pinkish in color. Its base forms a circular bulge, more prominent at the back of the penis, the crown of the glans. This is separated from the foreskin insertion by a circular groove, the glans neck.
Its apex is pierced by a sagittal slit of around 7 mm, the external ostium of the urethra.
Its urethral surface features a median groove joining the neck and the external urethral ostium, and giving insertion to the foreskin brake. Anatomy of the male genitalia :
*The Verge and clinical and surgical implications:*
*The envelopes of the penis form a cylindrical fold around the glans, the prepuce, which is arranged in a sleeve around the glans. Circumcision involves excision of the foreskin.*
*There is no cleavage plane at the level of the balanoprepucial sulcus, which is why the coronal incision during penile fracture surgery should be made 3 mm behind the sulcus.*


**Figure 1 Structural diagram of the penis (a=showing the body plus root of the penis and its relationship to the ischiocavernosus and bulbo cavernosus muscles; b=cross-section).**

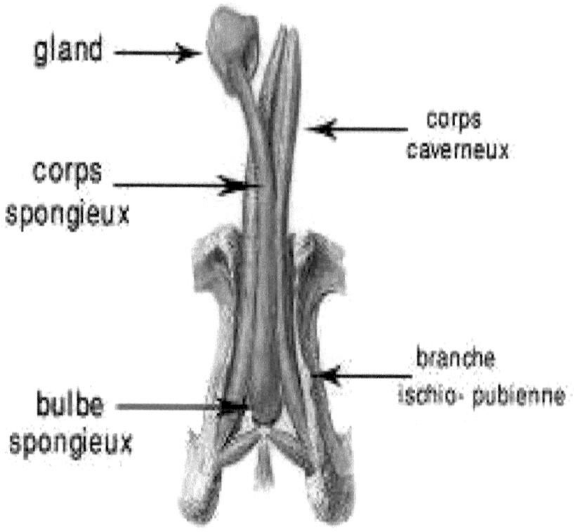



Fig 1 a

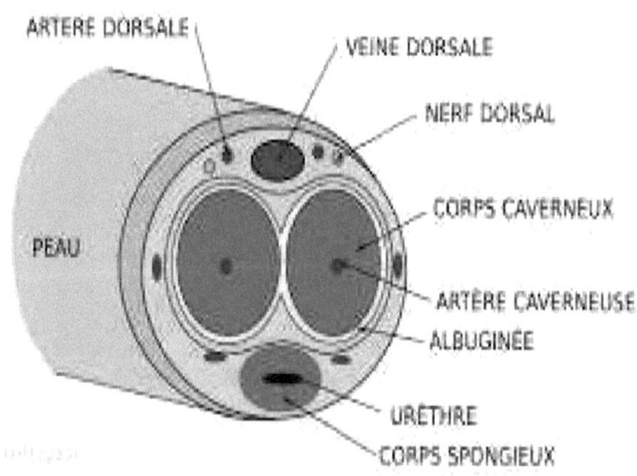



Fig 1 b

***Rod structure***

*B- d. **Vascularization, innervation and lymphatic drainage of the penis :***

*A.	Arteries:*

1.   Deep artery of the penis: derived from the internal pudendal artery. It runs along the axis of the corpus cavernosum. It gives rise to the helical arteries that open into the cavernous sinuses.

2.   Dorsal arteries of the penis:

Also originate from the internal pudendal artery. Run along the back of the penis on either side of the deep dorsal vein. They anastomose at the level of the glans neck, forming an arterial circle with branches for the glans, prepuce and prepuce frenulum. They give rise to circumflex arteries of the penis for the corpus cavernosum and the corpus spongiosum.

3.   Bulbar artery: directed to the spongy bulb.

4.   The urethral artery: vascularizes the cancellous urethra and the anterior part of the corpus spongiosum.

5.   Superficial arteries of the penis: These come from the external pudendal arteries, branches of the femoral artery. They supply the skin of the penis

***Arterial vascularization of the penis, showing the pudendal nerve in the yellow background***

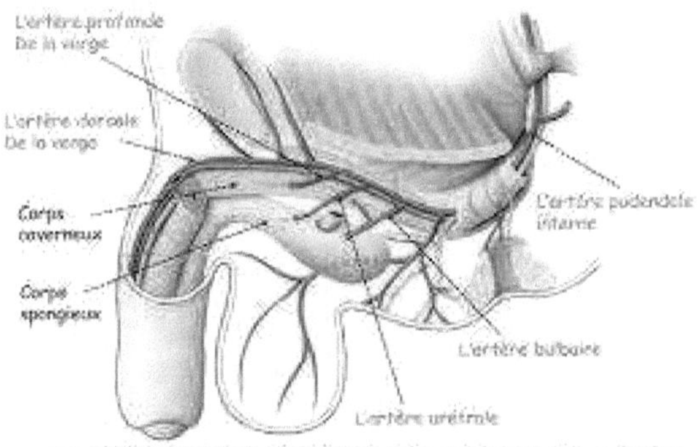


***Veins:***

*a. Veins of the erectile bodies :*

1.   The cavernous veins are drained by emissary veins either in the

circumflex veins, which join the deep dorsal vein of the penis, or in the bulbar veins, or directly in the internal pudendal veins.

2.      The deep dorsal vein of the penis: Drains the glans penis and the free part of the corpora cavernosa. It runs along the back of the penis under the deep penile fascia, joining the right and left internal pudendal veins; these veins also drain into the retro pubic plexus.

3.      Cavernous body roots:

drain directly into the retro pubic venous plexus or internal pudendal veins.

4.      Corpus spongiosum: drained by circumflex veins into the deep dorsal vein of the penis, and by bulbar veins into an internal pudendal vein.

*B.      Skin veins :*

Drain into the dorsal superficial penile vein, which can either join the external pudendal veins, tributaries of the great saphenous veins, or drain into the periprostatic plexus.

***Venous and arterial vascularization, taking innervation into account figure 2( a and b)***

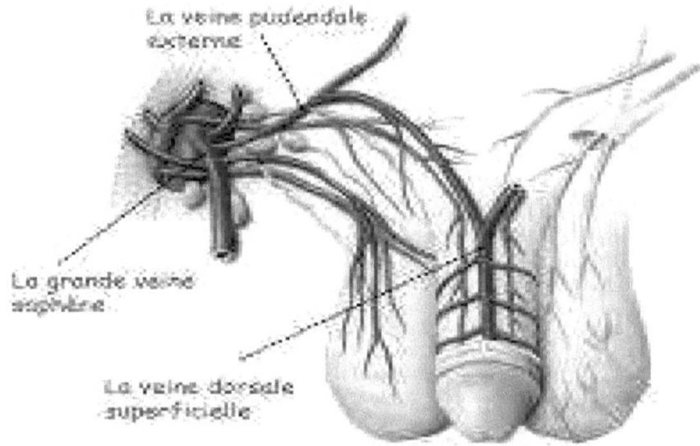


*a*

***Fig2: Vascularization showing the helical aa, emissary vv and circumflexes of the penis (Pierre Kamina)***

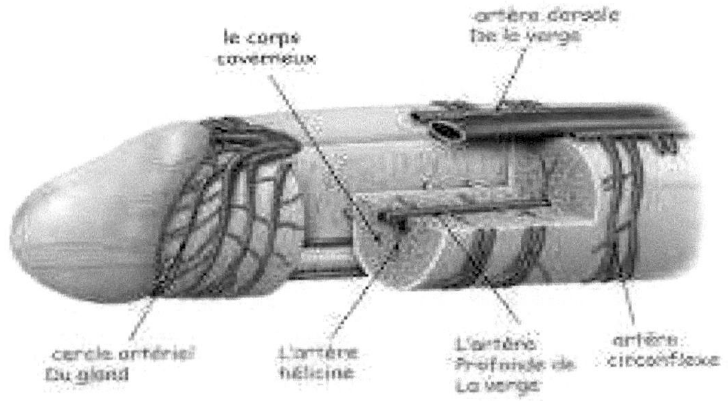



*b*

***Innervation of the penis:***

\-	*The vegetative system, comprising the SPS from the sacral medulla (S1, S2, S3, S4) and the SS from the dorsolumbar medulla (D10- 12).*

\-	*The somatic system also originates from the sacral medulla, responsible for penile sensitivity via the dorsal nerve of the penis and perineal motricity (ischio cavernosus and bulbo spongiosus muscles).*

\-	*EKARDT's erector nerve (a nerve originating from the somatic system and*

\-	*parasympathetic)*

\-

***Figures A and B: diagram of the innervation of the penis***

*A- A diagram showing the different routes and their centers*

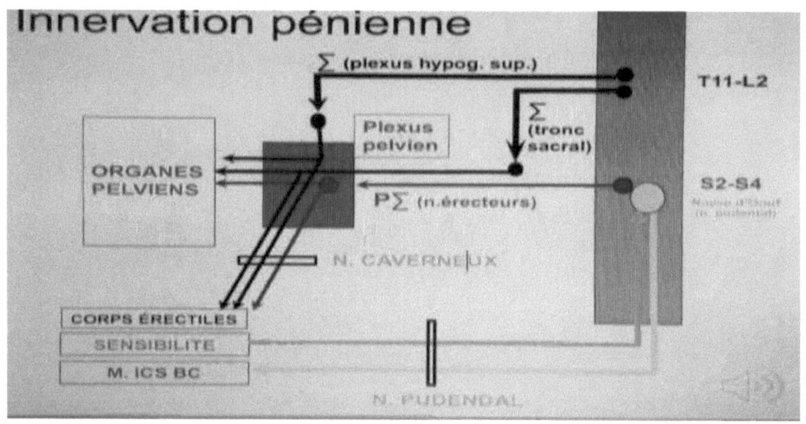



*B - anatomy*

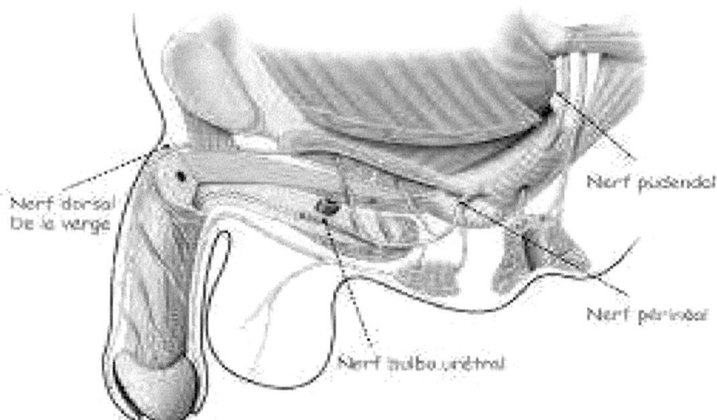



### C- Physiological reminder of the erection

It responds to the dynamic phenomena of the erectile bodies and to neurohormonal control.

### 1/ Erectile body dynamics

### a) Biodynamically defined erection at maximum pressure between 100 and 120 mm Hg

It begins with penile tumescence (lacunar filling), followed by rigidification to allow penetration, reinforced by the contraction of striated muscles attached to the erectile bodies.


-    **Tumescence:maximum pressure reached at 50mhmhg**:allows the penis to reach maximum volume as the cavernous lacunae are filled by two cavernous arteries (branch of the internal pudendal artery) branching off towards the areolae,

*All locoregional atheromatous conditions may be responsible for impotence due to a lack of*

-    Filling is only possible when the trabecular smooth muscle cells relax and close the areola in a flaccid state, under the dominance of sympathetic tone.

-    **Rigidification**: maximum pressure reached at 100 to 120 mm Hg is linked to blockage of venous drainage by compression of the emissary veins against the inner surface of the albuginea, with intra-cavernous blood pressure reaching its maximum. Despite the blockage of penile blood flow, oxygenation of intra-penile structures remains sufficient if the erection lasts less than 3 hours.


*b / Return to flaccidity (PDE5)*

When desire falls, the dominant sympathetic tone reduces the arterial blood supply to the areolae, allowing a drop in cavernous pressure which lifts the venous drainage blockage. Lacunar emptying then takes place via the emissary veins, which cross the albuginea, joining the circumflex veins surrounding the corpora cavernosa and draining into the deep dorsal vein of the penis.

Arterial input and venous output thus balanced, ensuring normal cellular metabolism of intra-venous components

*Figure 4: Diagram of erectile physiology and visualization of neuro-mediator effects*

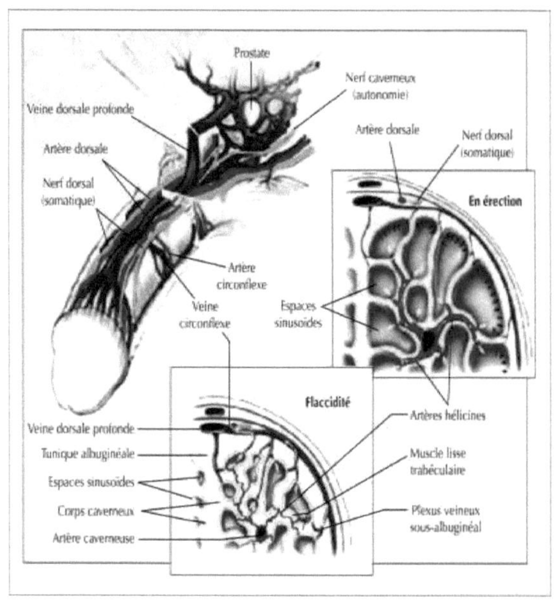

*a)      Microstructure in flaccid and erect state*

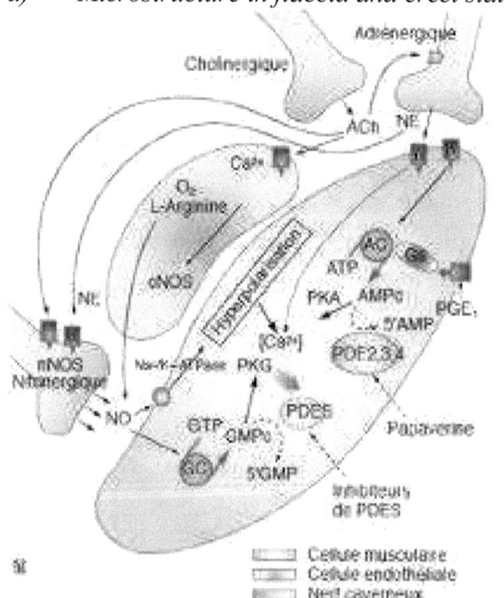

*b)      neuromediators and muscle cells*

## 2. Neurohormonal control

_ somatic innervation, as seen in the anatomical review of the penis, comes from the sacral medulla (S1, S2, S3, S4), which provides sensitivity via the dorsal nerve of the penis and motor function (ischio and bulbo cavernous muscles) via the perineal nerve.

Somatic innervation **is** involved in erection, particularly of the reflex type. Tactile palpation of the penis leads to the parasympathetic sacral centers, generating parasympathetic (vegetative) stimulation via Eckardt's erector nerves and motor stimulation via the internal pudendal nerves.

*- The vegetative innervation of the sympathetic and parasympathetic corpora cavernosa* is psychogenic (under cortical control).

+ Parasympathetic fibers arise directly from the anterior face of the sacral roots and give rise to Eckardt's erector nerve, which joins the cavernous nerve via the inferior hypogastric plexus.

+ Sympathetic fibres originate from the dorsolumbar medulla (D12-L2) and join either the internal pelvic and pudendal nerves, or the cavernous nerve via the superior and inferior hypogastric plexus.

## PHYSIOLOGICAL IMPLICATIONS OF THE GEGETATIVE SYSTEM

*In the corpus cavernosum, smooth muscles associated with the conjunctival skeleton trabecular :*

-        *Can contract and cause closure of the areolae, leading to flaccidity on sympathetic action (at rest, the penis is under sympathetic control).*

-        *Relaxation, (opening and filling of the areoles, penile expression) is under the action of the parasympathetic and the action of vasoactive substances such as NO, prostaglandin, expulsion of calcium from muscle cells under the action GMPc produces the GMP of NO activation, this phenomenon leads to relaxation and opening of the sinusoids*

*Superior control Physiological implications*

*Superior control is provided by the hypothalamic supraoptic nucleus in the anterior wall of the third ventricle, which receives information from Broca's limbic lobe: the anatomical basis of libido, itself subject to olfactory, visual, auditory and tactile sensory stimulation.*

*The supraoptic nucleus is also closely linked to the pituitary gland and influences its secretions.*

*Stimulation of libido leads to sympathetic inhibition and parasympathetic stimulation and release of vasoactive substances (NO, PGE1).*

*Ejaculation or the fall of desire leads to the return of sympathetic tone through the release of PD5*

*Androgenic hormone impregnation is essential for erection*
**D- ETIOPATHOGENY**

Micro-architecture of the penis

It is made up of transverse collagen fibers and elastic fibers aligned longitudinally.

Collagen fibers prevent the penis from expanding too much during erection, and allow it to return to the resting position during detuming. The albuginea of the corpora cavernosa is 2mm thick when the penis is at rest, but can thin to 0.25-0.50mm during erection, and becomes vulnerable to sudden mechanical stress (15 ), rupturing above 1500mmHg pressure (16).

Under the effect of a sudden overpressure, the brittle albuginous undergoes a rupture, these phenomena are ;

- Vigorous vaginal intercourse in 30-50% of Western countries (11) called coite faux pas (context: misfortune or sexual athleticism)

- Sexual intercourse in an upright position when the partner suddenly falls, causing a sudden curvature (4, 9, 21, 22).

- Untimely manipulation of the erect penis is much more common in the Middle East (attempt at concealment).

- Masturbation Doggy style positions :

- Sodomy 30% and Andromics 20%.

This phenomenon leads to the formation of anatomical-pathological lesions:

- Transverse, unilateral rupture of albuginea and cavernous tissue on the right in 75% of cases.

- Proximal and dorsal (16 19 2143 50 66 81) most often during false coites steps and very rarely distal (10) in 86.8% for Zargooshi (22) and 55.6% for El

Taher .dans la série de Zargooshi la majorité des lésions se siège à la partie proximale et dorsale

-       Urethral rupture 20-38% Western ( 3% Persian Gulf and Japan). More common if bilateral corpora cavernosa fractured (12 49 61 74), may be complete or partial ( 6 9 28 30 49 59).

-       Rupture of the suspensory ligament

-       Vascular rupture

Rupture of the albuginea of the corpus cavernosum may be localized, but can also extend to the urethra.

look for associated lesions. Injury to the urethra is more frequent in bilateral

fractures of the corpora cavernosa, and most often manifests itself as

urethrorrhagia. Total rupture of the urethra occurs in 2% of cases [3].

Clinical presentation is usually typical. Questioning should include a search for

the following:

_ Mechanism of the accident (circumstances are often difficult to ascertain) ;

hearing and/or cracking sensation; _ immediate detumescence of the penis; _ urethrorrhagia leading to suspicion of urethral rupture.

Partner ;

_ Appearance of localized pain in the penis (no correlation between severity of fracture and intensity of pain)

pain). A haematoma may extend in the shape of a pinna over the pubis, creating

the classic eggplant i m a g e , with the penis facing away from the lesion.


*Figure 5 Aspect of an eggplant-shaped penis in the second patient: penis facing away from the lesion*

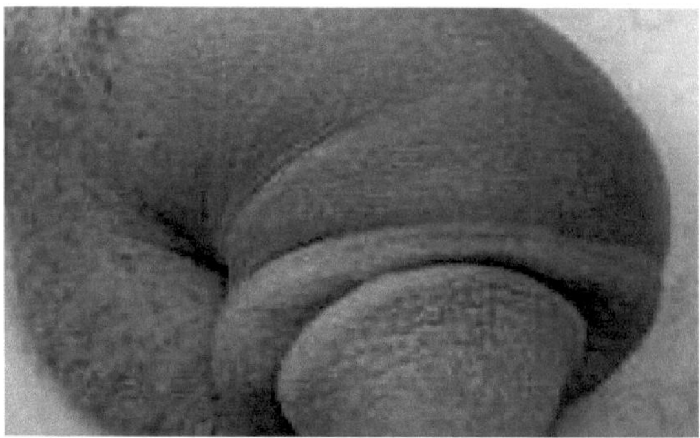

*Figure 6 Aubergine aspect of the second patient's penis: penis facing away from the lesion*


## *E- EPIDEMIOLOGY*

*AGE*

It is most often a pathology of the young, with an average age of 28.9. For Eke (7), this can be explained by the high level of sexual activity at this age. Ishikawa confirms in his series that 81% are between 20 and 50 years of age, when sexual intercourse is more frequent (11). Anecdotally, 73% of the men in Nouriy's series were unmarried (12).

### *Frequency:*

The Iranian series is the largest Zargooshi series, with 172 cases(22);

Only 185 aces had been reported up to 1985 (13).

In 1991, Mansi (15) counted 235 cases, including 14 in his own series, and in 1998, Mydlo (28) reported 250 cases in the Anglo-Saxon literature.

The number described in the 1935-2001 literature was 1,642 CAS (21).

*Distribution :*

It's a trauma that can be found all over the world, but there are certain areas of the globe where we still see more:

- the Middle and   Near East, and North Africa (21, 22). In Iran, ZAAGOOSHI (22) averaged one case per week in the emergency department of the university hospital,  representing 0.63% of urological emergencies.


## *F- DIAGNOSIS :*

### *Interrogation: ( 22,*

Questioning will attempt to establish the exact circumstances in which the injury occurred, and how long it took for the patient to seek medical attention after the trauma, which is generally less than 24 hours. DR Zarghooshi found 21.5 hours in his series and Muentener).

Trauma to an erect penis, accompanied by a sudden cracking sound that can be heard by the patient or partner (10, 11, 12,13, 14) , followed by detumescence and pain (15 ,16)

The appearance of a hematoma forming the wings of the auricle is a sign of a proximal, high-grade fracture.

In some cases, the patient may consult a doctor at a stage of curvature of the erect penis, or for ED (erectile dysfunction) revealing forms seen late in the complication phase, or for the presence of fibrosis (15).

Urethro-cavernous or urethro-cutaneous fistula or dysuria due to urethral stenosis (15,16 ,17)

Clinical examination:

Clinical examination reveals an aubergine-shaped penis (hematoma and edema progressively appear), *see figure 5, with the penis deviated, with its back to the lesion.*

Palpation can sometimes reveal a depression when the hematoma is not as large in front of the lesion (21).

*The Rollin sign identifies the fracture site (the clot that forms at the fracture site is palpable under the skin of the penis rolling over it (24)).*


***Figure 7: Typical appearance of a fractured penis (eggplant)***

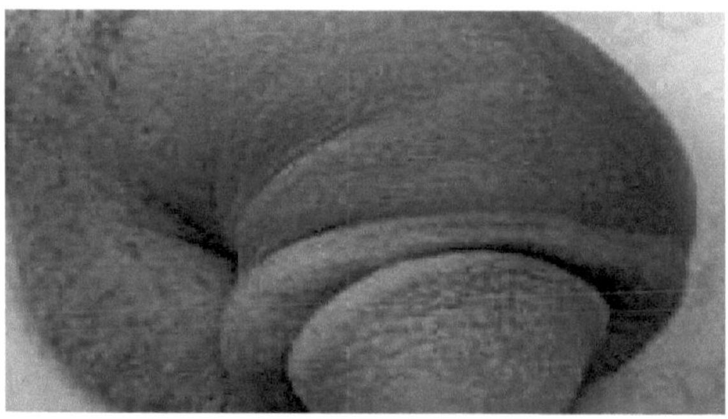

*Aspect of a preoperative fracture of the penis seen at 5 o'clock following a false coitus step at HMIMV Rabat in 2O2O in a 21-year-old patient: typical eggplant aspect and backing his lesion.*


***Figure 8: Fracture of the penis classified as type 3 or grade 3 in one of our patients.***

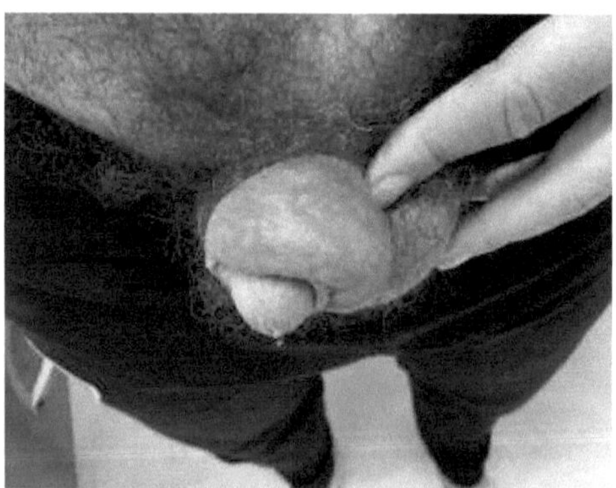

*Fracture of the penis with expansion of the haematoma onto the pubis on 05/2023, classified as type 3 (damage to the cavernous and proximal bodies, no associated lesions: butterfly wings).*

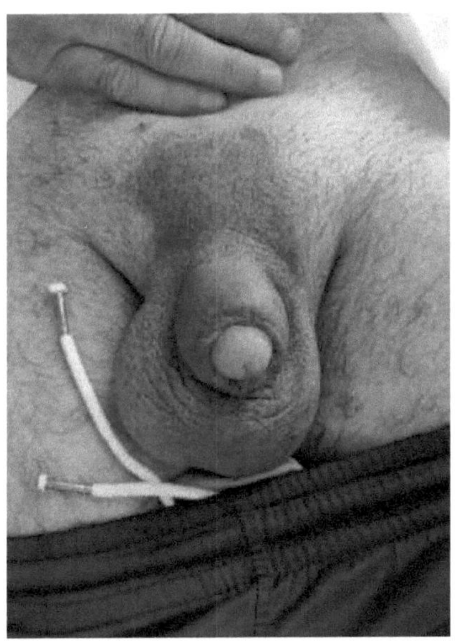

*Complementary examination (16, 21, 22, 23, 24,28, 29)*

The diagnosis of a fracture of the penis is based on a number of arguments gathered from the questioning and clinical examination. However, imaging plays an important role in determining the location of the lesion and the collaterals.

1 - Contribution of ultrasound :

High-frequency ultrasound, 7.5 MHz superficial probe: color Doppler verifies the integrity of the arterial and venous network of the penis

It is the first-line emergency examination, inexpensive, accessible and non-invasive, providing rapid information on the site and size of the lesion and collaterals (21, 22). However, it does have its limitations (small fracture difficult to see, large haematoma in front of the lesion, plus subcutaneous oedema hampering interpretation, or an operator unaccustomed to this type of lesion). Fractures are sometimes difficult to detect in the distal part of the penis for reasons of contrast and echogenicity between different tissues (24).

Ultrasound can be used to diagnose an albuginea defect.

An echogenic collection: reveals a hematoma, no Doppler signal in the hematoma

**2- *Contributions of cavernography (16, 21, 24 28) :***

It is a simple examination that can be performed with or without anaesthesia, indicated for all patients, while others reserve it for situations that are seen late: more than 24 hours in order to choose surgical or conservative treatment.

***Complications :***

a)      Priapism

b)      Allergic reaction

c)      Cavernous body fibrosis due to PDC extravasation

d)      Infection

e)      This examination may aggravate the post-traumatic hematoma and remains radiating and painful (24).

Contraindications are identical to IVUS 3- Contribution of MRI (24):

In this traumatic pathology, MRI provides a promising and encouraging result (10 25), and this examination has its place in the assessment of penile cancer extension and apyronia disease.

BOUBON reports in a study where he compared the sensitivity in penile fractures between ultrasound and MRI. MRI was superior with 100% sensitivity (25)

It's a costly examination, with limited availability, especially in emergencies, which would lengthen treatment times.

Technique: the patient is positioned supine, with the penis maintained in a vertical position, giving a penis close to erection and allowing correct examination of the proximal and distal parts, thus avoiding an artificial erection on a fractured penis.

A fracture line on the albuginea is seen as a hypo signal showing a solution of continuity in T1 and undetected in T2 ()

-       Subcutaneous hematoma seen in T1 rather than T2

\-     The intracavernous hematoma is well seen in T2, especially in T1 after injection of ganodium.

\-     The urethral mucosa is viewed with an early hyper-signal to see its course and discover any mucosal breaches.

*MRI: Classification into four grades;*

\-     *Type 1 Unilateral, single distal lesion, less than 20mm.*

\-     *Type 2 Unilateral, single lesion, distal, greater than 20mm.*

\-     *Type 3 Bilateral and/or multiple and/or proximal lesion.*

\-     *Type 4 Lesion associated with a ureteral wound*

*4-*     Place of retrograde urethrocystography (21,22, 24 ):

*UCRM*: is an examination most often used to diagnose urethral rupture in addition to corpora cavernosa rupture, and can sometimes transform partial urethral rupture into complete rupture ().

False positives have been reported in cases of urethral compression by penile hematoma (1,21,28,30,).

UCRM (21) in all patients presenting with urethrorrhagia prior to surgery, **Zargooshi** (22) also performs this examination in cases of dysuria, hematuria associated with rupture of the corpus cavernosum.

If there is no extravasation of contrast medium, a preoperative fibroscopy should be performed (25).

*E- TREATMENT*

The first case of a surgically treated fracture was reported in 1936 by FETTER (27); 24 years later in 1957 FERNSTROM supported this procedure (26).

At present, the reference treatment is still surgery, despite the conservative method which is sometimes requested either in the context of refusal of surgery or when MRI is performed, no lesion, but presence of an infiltrate, a small haematoma, and preservation of erection( 12, 21, 22, 23 ,24 ).

**A- Principles (12, 21, 22, 24, 25)**

a-     Principles of conservative treatment: remember that this is not a reference treatment. It consists of applying an ice bladder or a compress soaked in ice serum, and prescribing analgesics and anti-inflammatories, antibiotics and benzodiazepines.

b-      Principle of surgical treatment

A literature review was carried out, and the results were in favor of early management once the diagnosis of cavernous body fracture is accepted, with antibiotics prescribed for 08 days (27).

1)      Anesthesia Treatment can be carried out u n d e r  local, spinal or general anesthesia.

Some authors support the elective approach under local anaesthesia, allowing patients to return home the same day (24).

2)      Approach:

Several routes are possible, namely coronal incision 2-3mm from the balanopreputial sulcus with complete decantation, allowing a global view of the corpora cavernosa and the corpus spongiosum, but exposing the patient to complications such as infection, oedema and skin necrosis with a frequency of 14 to 25%. For ALBANY, the coronal incision is unique, as in the vast majority of cases the lesion is proximal.
(20) and has side effects (damage to superficial nerves leading to hyposensility of the penis).
It is particularly important to preserve the prepuce in the case of urethral involvement, for a possible **FERGAGNY** uretroplasty (28).

Longitudinal, lateral incision of a corpus cavernosum opposite the lesion enables an elective approach without risk of comorbidities, but at the cost of an unsightly scar.

The scrotal incision can be made at the scrotal level, and degrafting is also possible by this route for proximal fractures.

*Intraoperative image of a fractured penis in a 21-year-old in 2020 HMIM V Rabat who underwent an elective incision.*

**Figure 9- Type 1 fracture**

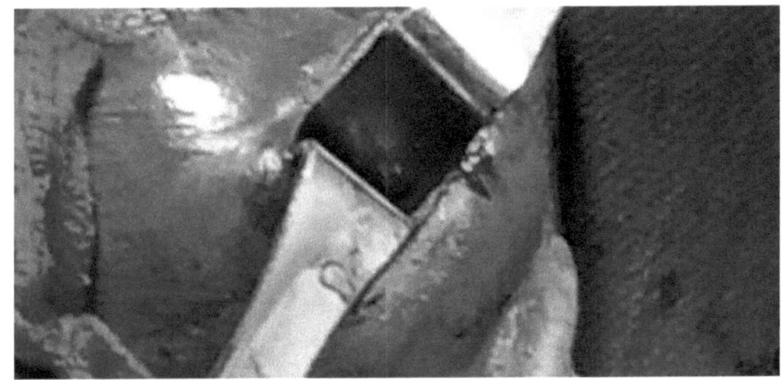

Figure: per op a

# BEFORE BANDAGING

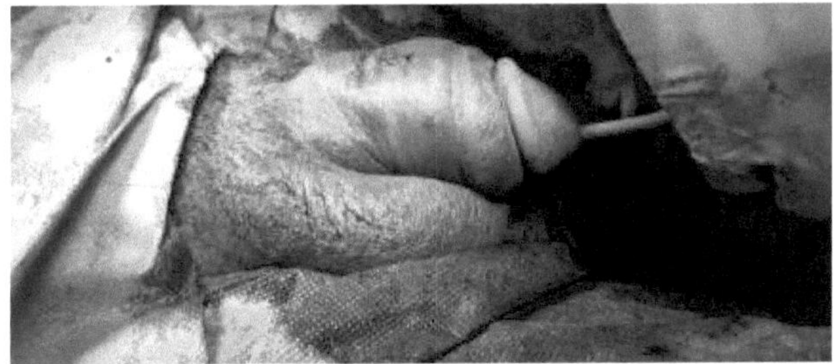

b

# After the operation

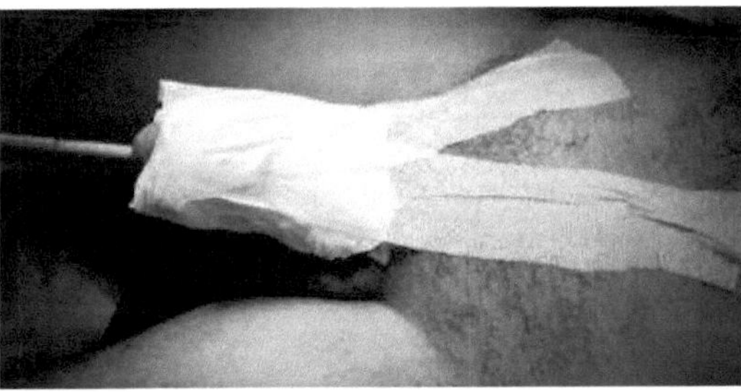

c

*Figure 10: Grade 3 surgery on figure 4 (A= lesion exposure and B= after lesion closure)*

*A        B*

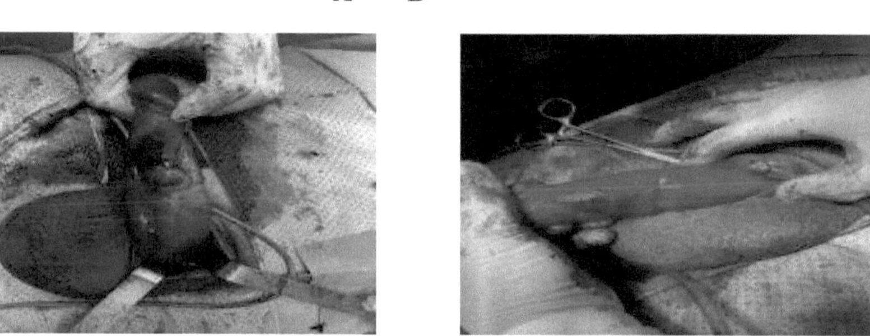

*Figure- 11 Intraoperative image of type 3 verge fracture in O5/2023*

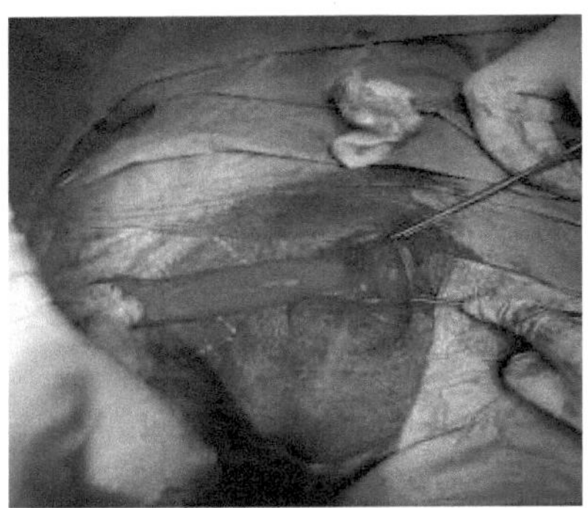 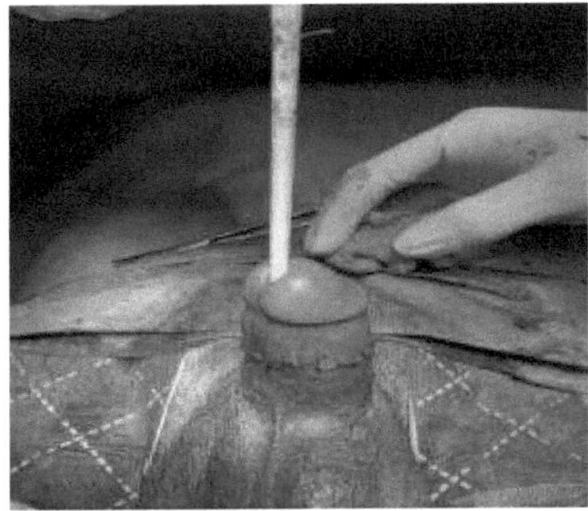

### 3 - *In case of associated urethral lesion :*

In **situations where there is an associated urethral lesion** (observed above all in the case of ventral and bilateral fracture of the penis), **FORGGNY** (28) recommends exploration of the spongy body, with ureteroscopy performed preoperatively for diagnostic and therapeutic purposes.

**4- Drainage**: no indication despite practice by some authors

Dressing: in order to control any ischemia or necrosis at an early stage, good practice recommends, according to the literature, bandaging the penis over a vesical probe, leaving the glans bare.

**5- Post-operative management:** to minimize the risk of recurrence and avoid early post-operative erection, **MYDLO** suggests prescribing **diethylstilbesterol** (28,29).


## F- VASCULAR ASSESSMENT AFTER SURGERY FOR FRACTURED PENIS

### Echo-doppler after injection of 10microg prostaglandin E1 early surgical position

*1)   Measurement*
-   *Peak arterial systolic velocity in the cavernous artery (PVS) Result:*
*increase in systolic velocity and positive diastolic appearance, see diagram*
-   *End-diastolic arterial velocity ( EDV)*
*Result: drop in diastolic flow with diastolic wave notch*
-   *Vascular resistance index equal to PSV - EDV /PSV*
*2)   **Results :***
*PSV less than 25 cm/second after injection of PE1 at 5mn is arterial insufficiency*
***VEINAL INSUFFICIENCY** (caverno-occlusive dysfunction): defined as **PSV** greater than 25 cm/sec and **EDV** greater than 5 cm/sec, accompanied by rapid detumescence*
-   ***IR less than 0.75***

*__Figure 12__: See the surgical post-exploration tracing diagram, which even fits into some EDs.*

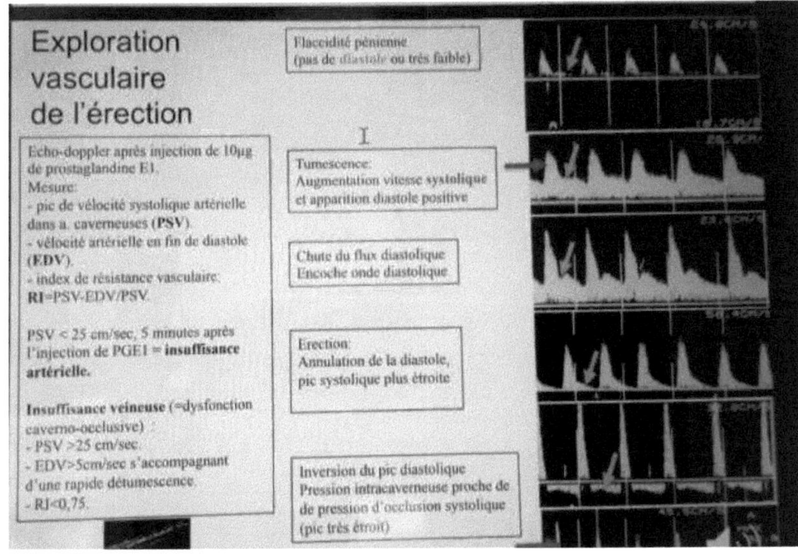



## VASCULAR EXPLORATION IN POST-SURGICAL SITUATIONS

## *MATERIALS AND METHOD*

A retrospective, descriptive study extended over 04 years was conducted between 2020- 06 / 2023 at the Hôpital Militaire d'Instruction Mohammed V Rabat Service d'Urologie.

Patients with penile fractures were included.

The databases used were the department's hospitalization register, the emergency room report register and medical records.

The parameters studied were age, circumstance of onset, reason for consultation, mechanism of onset, physical examination data, time to onset, treatment instituted, postoperative follow-up and sexual function after treatment. For all numerical variables, a mean was calculated and extremes defined.

At the end of our survey, 06 patients were included ***Table 1: Age distribution of***

***patients N= 06***

| Age groups years | number | Frequency |
|---|---|---|
| 20 à 29 | O1 | 16.66 |
| 30 à39 | O1 | 16.66 |
| 40 à 49 | O2 | 33.33 |
| 50à 59 | O1 | 16.66 |
| 60 à 69 | O1 | 16.66 |

The most represented age group is 40 to 49.

*No. 2 Distribution of patients by mechanism of occurrence*

*N=06*

| mechanisms | no | Frequency |
|---|---|---|
| Faux pas de coite | O5 | 73.33 |
| Forced handling | O1 | 16.66 |

The coite faux pas is most represented in our series

*N° 3 Distribution of patients b y   topography and anatomical site of lesion*

*N= O6*

| Body cavernous /uni or bilateral | number | Frequency |
|---|---|---|
| C body left and side | 02 | 66.66 |
| Bilateral proximal and dorsal | 04 | 33.33 |
| Total | 06 | 1OO % |

Involvement of the left corpus cavernosum was more marked in our series (06 cases out of 06), with bilaterality in 04 cases (66.66%).

**N° 4 Distribution of patients according to time between fracture and emergency visit**

N= O6

| Duration in hours | Number | Frequency |
|---|---|---|
| 5 Hours | 02 | 33 .33 |
| 7 Hours | 01 | 16.66 |
| 8 Hours | 01 | 16.66 |
| 27 Hours | 01 | 16.66 |
| 315 hours (15 days) | 01 | 16.66 |
| Total | 06 | 1OO % |

The delay is 05 hours for two of our patients The maximum delay is 15 days for one patient.

*N° 5 Distribution of patients by length of hospital stay*

*N= 06*

| Duration in hours | number | Frequency |
|---|---|---|
| 24 Heures | O1 | 16.66 |
| 12 Hours | O5 | 83.33 |
| Total | 06 | 100    % |

Hospital stay: 12 hours for 05 patients

24H for a patient due to delay before consultation about 15 DAYS

*Table n= 6: Distribution of patients according to post-operative outcome*

*N= 06*

| results | number | frequency |
|---|---|---|
| Good result | 05 | 83,66% |
| Bad result | 01 | 16,34 % |
| **TOTAL** | **06** | **100%** |

In this study, only one complication was diagnosed postoperatively at D30, marked by a curvature of the penis.

*According to Clavien and Dindo's complication concerning the mode of hospitalization, duration of hospitalization, mode of patient discharge and patient revisits at d15, d30 at 03months and at 6-months at the consultation, we found only one complication (a curvature of the penis).*

*No ED, urinary or infectious complications*

## *DISCUSSION*

The fracture of the penis has been observed for over 1,000 years by Abul Kassem in Coudoue, and was first documented in 1925 (16).

**A- Epidemiology B-**

### a- Morocco's place in the world - age

It is a rare pathology of young adulthood, and Eker believes it can be explained by the high level of sexual activity at this age (21).

A worldwide distribution has enabled us to retain the following:

Morocco in third place with 226 cases up to 2001, behind Iran in second place with 240 cases, and North America with 250 cases (USA and Canada).

The series of nouri in Morocco reports 56 cases in 08 years, then the latest largest Moroccan series published in 201O in Marrakech also reports 56 cases in 7 years of DR Saïd ARZA

In our series, among the 06 patients, the age group most represented was 40-49, i.e. 33.33%.

All these series report a predominance of young adults despite a divergence in etiology.

In our series, the average age of discovery was 32 years.

Yapanoglu (35) reported in 2009 in Turkey a mean age of 35.5 years in a population of 42 patients.

Zargooshi in Iran (22) in 2000, average age 26 in a population of 172 PATIENTS

Koudar (20) in the USA in 2008, a mean age of 39 years in a population of 08 patients.

**b-    Martial status**

In our series, 66.67% were unmarried and 33.33% married, in line with the data in the literature and with that reported in the series by DR said (21) in Marrachech in 2010, where 83% were unmarried and 17% married.

This high frequency can be explained by inexperience and increased vigor among young people.


## c-    Etiologies

Among the etiologies identified in the literature as possible causes of corpora cavernosa fractures, two were identified in our series: false coitus (83%) and forced manipulation of the erect penis (16.66%).

Our series differs from that of DR Saïd (21) and Nouri (12), who report respectively 66.1% and 66% of forced manipulation and 8% and 7.1% of false coitus.

Zargooshi in his series reports 78.3% of forced manipulation and 7.9% on a population of 352 patients in

Margaris (34) EN 2008 in Greece reports on a population of 08 patients 100%. DE faux pas de coït which remains almost comparable to our series


## d-    Anatomical mechanisms and lesions

In our series, all fractures occurred on fully erect penises; bilateral lesions numbering (04) cases classified as type 4 were selected from a population of 06 patients and proximal e; a unilateral and average lesion a single case classified as type 1.

We found no ureteral involvement (which could be classified as type 4).

Zargooshi (22) reports in his series 91.2% proximal involvement, distal 3.2%, average 5.4%.

Chung in the China-Taiwan region 50% proximal, 30% moderate, 20% distal involvement

Abdel Nasser in a population of 24 patients reported 41.7% proximal, 50% average, 8.36% distal disease.

No urethral damage classified as type 4, which is very rare but exceptional.

e-    **Diagnostics**

In our series, the diagnosis is clinical and supplemented by penile ultrasound.

The circumstance of onset, pain, detumescence and the observation of the typical eggplant appearance is our diagnostic key and is found in all our patients.

Our diagnosis is in line with that in the literature, and is comparable with the various references (12, 13, 14, 15, 27).


f-    **Time elapsed before consulting the emergency department**

In our series, the minimum time is 05 hours and the maximum is 15 days, i.e. 360 hours in one patient.

The average consultation time is ......

According to the patient, this delay can be explained by shame.


g-    **Treatment**

Treatment was 100% surgical in our series, in line with the new recommendation in the literature and all the series we used as references, with elective incision in only one case out of 6 (1/6).

and 5/6 cases of coronal incision at 3mm balanopreputial groove

h-    **Suite opératoires**

the patients were reviewed at D15, D30 and at month (long term, six patients) in consultation

Only one of our patients had a curvature of the penis at an angle of 64° to the horizontal.

Our overall therapeutic results after this follow-up proved to be in line with the average of medical series ( 20, 22, 23, 24).

*Figure 13- The only complication found in our study series*

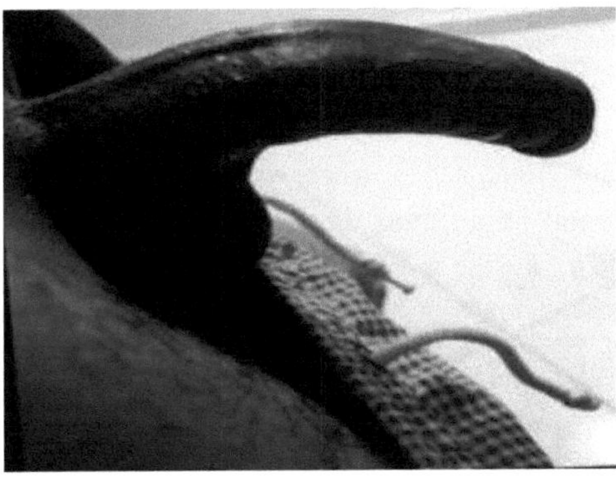

## i-      Comparison of some series with ours

Abdel Nasser (54) at six months, 95.8% rated good, penis curvature 4.2%, no sexual dysfunction

-       Dicel (45) average follow-up 21 months, good results=90.9%, no ED, no curvature
-       Mazaris (34) over 24 months of follow-up good result =100% good result
-       Fergany (28) in Cleveland, USA, over a period of 19 months 100% was classified as a good result.
-       Ours gave 83.34% good results and 16.66% bad results marked by curvature.

## *CONCLUSION*

Fracture of the penis is a rare pathology in young adults, with a variety of etiologies, but in our series, the most common cause was coital malunion, thus diverging from many Asian series, where the cause is by far forced manipulation of an erect penis, and joining the Western and North American series, where malunion remained by far the most common.

The fracture is audible to all our patients, and is accompanied by rapid detumescence of the penis, followed by a progressive hematoma, giving all our patients an eggplant appearance.

Diagnosis is clinical, but imaging such as MRI, ultrasound and cavernography can be very useful in pinpointing the exact location of the lesion and other associated lesions.

Treatment is surgical, involving either a coronal or elective incision, evacuation of the hematoma, watertight cavernorraphy and albinorraphy, and repair of any urethral damage during the same operation.

Medical treatment should be avoided, as it often leads to complications. Patients should be reviewed in consultation.

***Only one complication was noted in our series, marked by a curvature of the penis, and the patient was taken back for straightening of the penis by plicature.***

**SUMMARY**

***Introduction***

Observed despite more than 1000 years by Abul Kassem in Coudoue, trauma to the penis with rupture of the corpus cavernosum was first described and published in 1925 (64). This is a rare trauma to an erect penis, which must be treated early to avoid complications.

***Patients and methods:*** a retrospective study conducted at HMIMV Rabat over 04 years from January 2020 to December 2023, identified a series of 06 patients admitted for traumatic rupture of the corpora cavernosa.

***Results:*** At the end of this study, unlike the Asian series, in the Near and Middle East, the coitus faux pas came out on top (83.37%) and forced manipulation on an erect penis (16.66%).

Grade III represents 73.33

This is a pathology of young adults, with an average age of 34, and a predominance of single subjects.

***Diagnosis:*** is clinical, thanks to careful questioning and physical examination.

The symptomatology, although stereotyped, is marked in our chronological series by

-Cracking noise in 100% of cases

- the 100% douteur

-100% detumescence

- the appearance of a 100% hematoma, sometimes spread out like butterfly wings

***creating the typical eggplant look.***
*Hematuria and acute urine retention are pathognomonic signs of urethral damage.*

No examination appears to be essential. And all our patients were treated *surgically (elective approach or coronal incision)* and the evolution was favorable in 83.66% of cases and a curvature of the penis 1 case 16.33%.

***Conclusion:*** early surgical management is the ideal way to offset the risks of postoperative functional complications.

*OPERATION SHEETS*

Name :

**First name :**                                              *tel*........................

**Age :**

**Martial status :**

**History:**

**Circumstances in which the trauma occurred Consultation time :**

**Clinical examination of the penis on admission**

-     Pain                                                  yes               no
-     Hematoma                                 yes               no
-     Curvature of the penis                yes               no
-     Uretrorrhagia                         yes               no
-     Acute retention of urine            yes               no

    **Assessment: ultrasound**                      yes             no MRI :

                                                              yes     no

                    Cavernography :                    yes            no

**Surgical treatment**

-     **Approach**       :                           elective            coronal

-     **Lesion characteristics :**

Right left
Unilateral                                Bilateral
Distal medium                 proximal

**<u>Grade or type :</u>**

Type1 Yes                     no

Type2 YES                   NO

| Type 3 | YES | NO |
| Type 4 | YES | no |

**Evolution :**

-     Duration :
-     Sequelae :     functional     aesthetic
-     Surgical revision: yes     no

# BIBLIOGRAPHIES

1.    Paparel P, Ruffion A. Corpus cavernosum rupture: technical aspects of management. Ann Urol 2OO6 :40 :267-272.

2.    Grima F, Paparel P, Devonnec M, Perrin P, caillot JL, Ruffion A, : Prises en charge des traumatismes des corps caverneux du penis .Prog Urol 2006.16 :12-18

3. Trye CB. Case of a rupture oh the corporosa cavernosa penis. Med com 1784- 1790 London;ii 158- 162

4.   Franck JP: De courandis Hominum morbis. Liber v, pars II, 1807 ;p 281

5.   Mott V: Laceration of the corpis cavernosum penis commonly called fracture of the penis illustrated by two cases. The ter New-York acad Med1847-; I: 99-103.

6.   Huguier: Complete rupture of the urethral canal, partial rupture of the corpus cavernosum, death. Bulletin de la société de chirurgie de parie, April 1853, iii514- 518.

7.   Eke N. Fracture of the penis: Br J Surg 2002; 89: 555-565

8.    Redi R, A case of penile fracture. J Urol 1926- ; 22/36-44

9.    Thomson RF. Rupture of the penis, J Urol 1954. 71:226.

10.    Fernstrom U. Rupture of the penis: report of one operated case and review of literature.

11.   ISHIKAWA T.FUJISAWA M. TAMADA. H INOUE T. SIHIMATANI    N: Fracture of the penis: nine cases with evaluation of reponded case in japon. Int. J. Urol, 2003; 10:257-260.

12. Nouri M. Koutani A. Tazi K. El khadir K. Ibn Attaya A. Hachimi M. Lakrissa A.Fracture of the penis in 56 cases. Prog Urol, 1998; 8; 542- 647.

13. Taha S A. Sharaya A. Kamal B A. Salem A A. Khwasa S: Fracture of the penis: surgical management. Int Surg, 1988: 73:63_64

14. Mansi M K. Emran M. El Mahrouky A. El Mateet M S: Experience with

penile fracture in Egypt: long term results of immediate surgical repair. J Trauma 1993; 35: 67- 70.

15.    Mydlo J H, Hayyeri M, Macchia R J,: uretrography and cavernography imaging in a small series of penile fracture: a comparison of surgical findings . Urology, 1998; 51: 616- -619.

16.    Asgari M A. Hosseni S Y, Safarinjad MR. Samadzadeh B. Bardideh A R: Penile fractures: evaluation, therapeutic approach and long term results. Urol, 1996; 155: 148-149.

17.    E l bahnasawy MS. Gomba M A. : Penile fractures :the successful dotcom of immediate surgical intervention. Int. J. Impot; Resp, 2000; 12: 273-277.

18.    Muentener M. Suter S . Hauri D. Sulser T: long term experience of surgical and conservative treatment of penile fracture. J. Urol, 2004; 172:576-579.

19.    Ganem J P., Kennely M J: Ruptured Mondor's disease of the penis mimicking penile fracture. J Urol, 1998.159: 13O2.

20.    Saïd ARZA. Fracture of the corpus cavernosum about 56 cases in the department of urology at the military hospital of Avicenne Marrachech extended over a period of 8 years from 01/01 /2000 and 31/12/ 2007

21.    Zargooshi J. Trauma as the cause of peronie's disease: penile fracture as a model of trauma. J.Urol 2004: 172:186-188.

22.    Manguin P. Pascal B. Cukier J: accidental urethral rupture during coitus. J Urol 1983, 89:27-34.

23.    François G. Philippe P. Marian D. Paul P. Jean-Louis C ; Alain R : Prise en charge des traumatismes des corps caverneux du penis ; Service de chirurgie Urologique et de transplantation rénale, service des urgences chirurgicales viscérales, center hospitalier LYON sud, Pierre Bénite, France. Prog en Urologie (2006) / 16-12-18.

25.    Cumming J. Jenkins JD: fracture of the corpora cavernosa and urethral during sexual intercourse. Br. J Urol 1991; 67: 327.

26.    Fetter TR. Gartman N: Rupture of the penis. Case report. Am J. SURG, 1936; 32: 371-372.

27.   Fergany A F. Angermeler KW.   Montag D K. Review of Cleveland, Clinic experience with penile fracture. Urology 1999;54: 352- 355

28.   Mydlo J H. Hayyeri M. Macchia JR: uretrography and cavernosography imaging in a small series of penile fracture: a comparisons with surgical findings. Urology 1998;51: 616-619.

29.   Mydlo J H: surgeon experiences with penile fracture. J Urol. 2001: 166: 526- 528

30.   Godec CJ .Reiser R Logush AZ The erect penis injury prone organ. J.Trauma; 1998:28: 124 -126

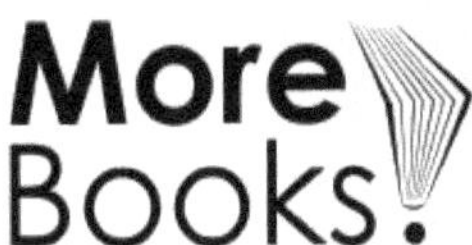


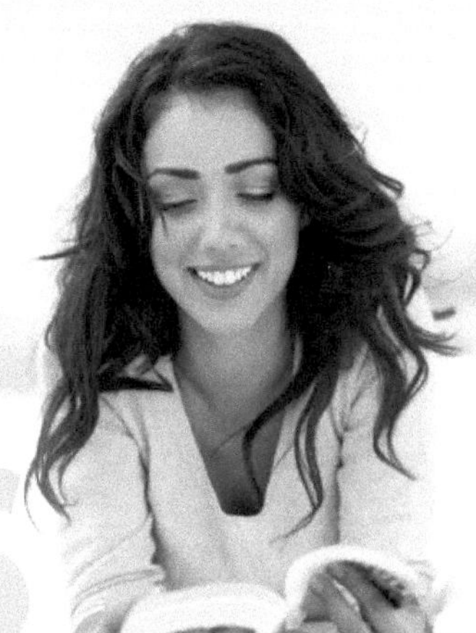


## I want morebooks!

Buy your books fast and straightforward online - at one of world's fastest growing online book stores! Environmentally sound due to Print-on-Demand technologies.

Buy your books online at
**www.morebooks.shop**

Kaufen Sie Ihre Bücher schnell und unkompliziert online – auf einer der am schnellsten wachsenden Buchhandelsplattformen weltweit! Dank Print-On-Demand umwelt- und ressourcenschonend produziert.

Bücher schneller online kaufen
**www.morebooks.shop**

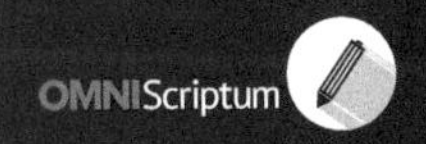

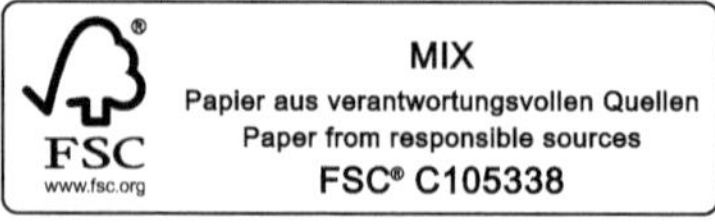


Printed by Books on Demand GmbH, Norderstedt / Germany